REPAIRING
the BENZO BLUNDER

A MOSAIC
of **RECOVERY**

A case of medical and pharmaceutical iatrogenesis

Marjorie Meret-Carmen, M.Ed.

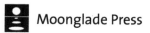 Moonglade Press

Moonglade Press
Publishing New Works by Uncommon Voices
Distributed by IngramSpark

ISBN: 978-0-692-90592-0
Library of Congress Control Number: 2017950103

Printed in the U.S.A.

Dedication

One of Judaism's most powerful and specific contributions to humanity is its Ethics of Responsibility, illustrated by social concepts of gratitude, philanthropy, kindness, and a mandate to "repair the world" known as Tikkun Olam. *Repairing the Benzo Blunder: A Mosaic of Recovery* is dedicated to that hopeful principle.

Contents

The Mandorela (Mandorla)

In the early 1990s while studying academic theology in Berkeley, California at the Graduate Theological Union, Pacific School of Religion I took courses from priests, rabbis, pastors, and mystics. I was also introduced to Kabbalistic Mysticism, an ancient philosophical language originally only available to married men over 40 and where I discovered the notion that the universe is comprised of "Four Worlds," levels of reality; that existence is multi-layered, and in dynamic flux from conception to manifestation.

While pondering the Kabbalistic concept of "Four Worlds" I designed something I called a "Mandorela," totally oblivious to the existence of the Vesica Piscis Mandorla,[2] an ancient symbol with many spiritual associations.

I have interpreted the Four Worlds as representing Vision, Education, Action, and Resolution.

Throughout this book I use the Mandorela to indicate a change of topic, chronology, or just a place to pause and think.

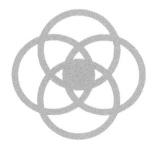

PILLS

They hand them out
Like candy
Little ones
Big ones
Round ones
Square ones
Triangles, some
Colors of the rainbow
Swallow this
Swallow that
...doesn't work?
Try this
...that doesn't work.
Try this
Side effects?
Even death?
Don't worry about it
Swallow this
Swallow that
While Pharma
Swallows the profits.

Part **I**

Intention

Since the mid-1950s, the proverbial "they" have been handing out pills like candy.

Want to lose that post-baby weight?
Have a few Dexedrine, (Amphetamines/Speed).

Want to have sex without getting pregnant?
Have some synthetic hormones to prevent ovulation. Imagine what that does to your natural feminine cycles.

Pregnant with a big baby and have a sore back?
Here, take a Percodan. Never mind how it will impact the baby's developing brain.

Unhappy?
Boy, do we have an array of antidepressants from which to choose. Don't worry about prematurely losing your neurons.

Anxious about something? Can't sleep?
We've got just the right thing for you.

A benzodiazepine!
This is one you should worry about!

My original intention in writing this book was to shed new light on a 60-year-old pharmaceutical travesty. In so doing, *Repairing The Benzo Blunder: A Mosaic of Recovery* became a much larger story; having grown beyond the journal I began writing in 2006 when my husband began exhibiting symptoms of dementia and I started having panic attacks and insomnia.

I hope my tale proves to be a helpful resource to physicians, families, and thousands of benzodiazepine (aka benzo) patients, who like me, made an uninformed and trusting choice that resulted in a four-year dependency on Lorazepam/Ativan. I encourage everyone to do their own study on the topic to reach their own conclusions.

Fragments on a Rising Moon

Monday, November 5, 2012, 4 am...

"Seriously, all I really want to do is die! Simple as that!"

"What the hell is happening to me?" I screamed into the bathroom mirror. An unkempt, haggard, emaciated version of myself stared back with swollen bloodshot eyes. My once long blond hair, now gray and stringy, my hands quivering as I tried to brush my teeth after what felt like hours on my knees hovering over the toilet, vomiting.

An Ativan Embryo

Throughout the winter of 2012, I lay on my side in bed, my legs drawn up embryo-like, my head propped up to see the laptop computer. My face as close to the screen as my husband's face used to be as we lay close to one another during the night – close enough to hear each other breathing, close enough to kiss.

Now, I curl the clumps of hair falling to my pillow into little balls, lining them up the base of the keyboard as I search for something or someone to tell me how to recover from Ativan's aftermath.

2006
Losing Words

I am in the kitchen making chicken salad, cutting the boiled organic chicken breasts into bite-sized pieces, Milton enters the room.

His signature blue, cashmere crew neck sweater and worn Levis (his adopted retirement garb) gives him the appearance of someone far younger than his 82 years.

He leans against the stainless steel refrigerator door and sighs. "Honey," he says matter-of-factly, "I am losing words."

My brilliant, eccentric, silver-haired fox of a husband is losing his Yale-educated marbles. Memories of my mother's neuro decline passed before my eyes. I look up and practically cut off my thumb, requiring twelve stitches at the nearby emergency room.

For someone as erudite as my husband, losing words was an alarm bell to be heeded. We immediately sought medical advice. Three neurologists told us three different things: first Parkinson's, then Alzheimer's, and then Lewy Body Dementia (LBD).[3] The only way to know for sure what was affecting his brain was via an autopsy.

Interestingly, as dementia's fog entered our lives, a different Milton surfaced. Without so many memories of disappointments, betrayals and stresses that go along with economic success, he began to enjoy the freedom of living in the moment, fully present in a way I doubt he had ever experienced; and with that, a new kind of tenderness and romance entered our lives.

Caring for him through these final years became a sacred task, requiring a triple dose of patience and total respect for his dignity. We were lucky, he didn't have to be "stored" somewhere, "like a nothing," as my mother would say after doing her volunteer piano playing (even at age 86) at local nursing homes.

I knew the protocol. What I did not know were the gifts awaiting me as I accompanied my husband through his declining years.

2007
Ativan, Welcome to My World

During one of Milton's medical appointments, I told his doctor I was having panic attacks and not sleeping well, having come to the realization the only outcome of dementia is death.

"Quite normal, given the circumstances," Dr. K. said casually pulling a prescription pad from the pocket of her crisp white smock. "Here, this will help."

The prescription: Ativan/1mg/100/ take as needed, up to 3mg per day.

I recognized the name because my husband had been per-scribed Ativan for years, and just about every tranquilizer that stumbled into the bio-psychiatric marketplace since the mid-1950s when he went into analysis with a Boston Freudian psychothera-pist. He also had five surgeries requiring general anesthesia in the last ten years. I wondered if these tranquilizers and anesthesia had anything to do with his evolving dementia.[4]

2009 – 2010

In Death We Did Part

"All that I have lost I find at every step and remember that I have lost it."
— ANTONIO PORCHIA

Tuesday, August 10, 2009, 3:00 a.m...

From our bedroom, I hear Milton's rasping breaths; no discomfort, no consciousness.
"Pneumonia," the Hospice fellow pronounces, placing a small patch of something on the back of my husband's neck. "He probably won't last the day," he says as kindly as possible.

He didn't.

I was numb, but not from any kind of shock. In the last year, my husband had declined into someone he would not have wanted to become.

I was numb because my emotions were masked by two years' worth of Ativan, leading up to that sea-change moment when the life we had created together flew out the window, along with my heart.

Concoctions

The rest of 2009 and 2010 remained a fog as I continued to mask the cellular grief, swallowing 3 mg of Ativan a day, never more. By the middle of 2010, I began gritting my teeth between doses. I sensed the Ativan was turning on me like a snake, causing increased anxiety, nausea, insomnia, and bouts of vertigo.

My brain was sending signals it wanted more, to stave off a new kind of anxiety, far more intense than the level that sent me to that first prescribing doctor in 2007. To make matters worse, I was not sleeping, sometimes for nights on end. I made poor decisions for the wrong reasons. Gradually I retreated from social encounters. All the while being told I was clinically depressed and just grieving the loss of my beloved. Their solution? I needed to see a psychiatrist. So, I did. She added to my pharma-cocktail, first Lexapro, then Zoloft (anti-depressants), Seroquel, Gabapentin, Celexa, and Trazodone. When one concoction made me more unraveled and nauseous, she switched me to another.

Finally, two serious bouts with vertigo sent me to Google, where I discovered not only that vertigo may be a side effect of a long-term relationship with a benzodiazepine, but also that just about every organ of our bodies is affected by these psychopharma concoctions.

When I persisted about stopping the Ativan, my psychiatrist Dr. T said she would help me taper off – very slowly, she emphasized. Because coming off a benzodiazepine too rapidly can cause seizures, and can actually kill you. However, she dismissed my suggestion, based on Professor Ashton's, Ashton Manual, that I switch to Valium before withdrawing.

I was at the mercy of her benzo knowledge – or lack of it.

Professor Heather Ashton

In doing research on my own, I found Professor Heather Ashton's bible of benzo awareness, withdrawal, and recovery, *The Ashton Manual*. Originally written in 2002, with updates and revisions through 2013.[5]

In 2007, when I swallowed my first 1 mg of Ativan – and got the first good night's sleep in weeks – I had no idea that, in the United Kingdom, Professor Ashton was speaking about the "extraordinary entanglement between drug companies and the medical profession."

This quote is both comforting and alarming.

"In some subjects the withdrawal syndrome can be protracted, lasting months or even years. Protracted symptoms include insomnia, depression and a variety of neurological and gastrointestinal symptoms which can be very distressing and may sometimes be permanent... So far there is no clear evidence of structural damage to the brain, though it has been suggested in some studies. Other studies have clearly shown long-lasting, cognitive deficits in long-term benzodiazepine users who have withdrawn."

Little did I know then, I would become one of the afflicted.

Gradually, I discovered it was not the fault of the doctors and other medical practitioners originally consulted on this benzo journey. They prescribed those little white pentagon-shaped pills to quell the obvious anxiety that accompanies the loss of a brilliant husband's mind and ultimately, his life. Their knowledge of psychiatric medications was limited to what the nicely dressed pharmaceutical sales representatives told them while handing out samples of the latest and greatest concoctions. My belief is these medical professionals were unaware of the damage those recipes could be doing to the same patients they intended to help.

At least at first.

Then something happened!

When competition and profit margins began to drive the engines good intentions got sideswiped, things chemical and ethical got out of control – especially when Psycopharma Goliath's marching band rolled into town. These medications tricked the brain to think all is well. When, in fact, all was not well. Early benzo warnings surfaced and were ignored by the worldwide medical community.

Hiding

Trapped in the pain/body
I am nothing
blessed with so much,
seeking peace in solitude
Will I ever be 'me' again?
I hide –
or am I in a womb
rebirthing myself?

"Every time I wake I understand how easy it is to be nothing."
— ANTONIO PORCHIA

Late Nights

Googling around cyberspace during one of my sleepless nights I discovered a social media forum, benzobuddies.org.[6]

There, over 15,000 members coping with being on or tapering off benzos, sharing their angst and triumphs, giving and receiving heartfelt support.

Anonymous friendships blossomed amongst a legion of benzo-wounded warriors, trapped in a relationship with a medication prescribed by their physicians. And they, like me, found those medications had turned on them, leaving so many of us howling late at night to the moon. No matter when I logged on there was someone ready to either commiserate or offer encouragement.

Yet, when I mentioned the forum to my primary care physician his condescending stare spoke volumes!

Friday, November 20, 2009, evening...

Scrambled Eggs

I lie here for hours, as, frame by frame, memories beat me from head to toe, scrambling my thoughts like eggs, whipping me from side to side. The right side of my body is coming apart, the shaking is constant. The gnawing in my back is vicious. The ache in my right knee persists; every step is a reminder. The belly quivers.

"Just do not move," I hear from within. I am shaking. Weeks of pain meds, narcotics. Time to forgive myself.

All the errors; all the terrors.

Sunday, November 22, 2009, morning...

Must
I must re-engage in life, a life that belongs to me
haul myself out of this deep well of grief of this pain/body
Tolle[7] *writes about.*
Move the oxygen and blood through my cells, exercise, eat,
pay bills.
Organize my world
As it is ...it is ... it is ...
Find my way out of this monkey mind.
I must get off of these drugs.

Tuesday, November 24, 2009, afternoon...

Jangled. Discombobulated. Undone. Apart at the seams.
I continue to shake. My left hand, my writing hand, out
of my control. Should I take an Ativan? Tramadol? Both? To
quell the quiver. If I don't, within hours the shaking starts, the
intense panic feeling. I am alone, something is wrong, I am
in agony. Days tick tock by, my head feels like a many-horned
dragon.

I had been working with Dr. M to withdrawal from the Ativan. Writhing on the floor wrapped in pillows and blankets to stop the shivering, I called him on his cell phone. He was in the car with his kids, I could hear them. "What should I do? Should I take an Ativan?" I asked. "Now Marjorie, there are no shortcuts" he answered.

Alone once more, I feel I have been dismissed.

Wednesday, November 25, 2009, evening...

Be Still-Know God-Be Still-Know God-Be Still-Know God
Divine intervention would be welcome right now.

Monday, November 30, 2009, morning...

Broken nerves and sinews
Constant nausea. My skin does not fit my body, it belongs to someone else.
What is the matter with me? What is making me so fearful?
I must force myself out of bed.
*Today I **will** leave the house!*

Thursday, December 31, 2009, evening...

Jagged
How harsh the holly
Wounds so deep
They do not bleed
In jagged fury
Scabs give way
to scars.

January–July, 2010

Fog
Grieving through Ativan's mask, I face the beginning of 2010 in a fog, a blur.
I have little recollection of the days, as they passed by.
All of a sudden, a year since he entered those "realms beyond reason" I read about.

Tuesday, August 10, 2010, evening...

Lost Year
One year tomorrow
seems like yesterday
lost year
now only pain.

Sludge

In early October, I underwent gall bladder surgery, the surgeon's solution to the gut-wrenching pain I was experiencing. "Gall bladder sludge. Needs to be removed. Don't worry, you won't miss it," I was told.

Now, five weeks later, I was packing for Boston to attend meetings at Mass General's Massachusetts Institute of Neurodegenerative Disease (MIND). I was scheduled to speak at a fundraiser, encouraging people to donate to this wonderful group of scientists trying to find the cures for neurodegeneration of all persuasions.

However, when I landed in Boston I again experienced the same gut-wrenching pain. I had to give my fundraising pitch from a wheelchair. After the speech was over I ended up in Mass General's emergency room. There, I was given a lot of drugs, and this is when I began to wonder if the Ativan had anything to do with my gall bladder sludge.

When I got home, I looked on benzobuddies for "benzodiazepines and gall bladder problems." There I found several noted instances of people having to have their gallbladder's removed.

Trouble

Toward the end of 2010, I knew I was in trouble. If I took more than the 1 mg of Ativan three times a day I was a zombie. If I didn't, I became an anxious, fear-filled, nauseous woman.

On November 18, I discovered an article written by Christopher Lane, Ph.D. stating:[8] "Psychiatrists have long known that benzodiazepines can cause brain damage."

In 2010, Britain's *Independent* newspaper published a bombshell for psychiatry and medicine. The country's Medical Research Council had sat on warnings 30 years earlier that benzodiazepines such as Valium and Xanax can cause brain damage.[9]

Nearly 11.5 million prescriptions for these drugs were issued in 2008 in Britain alone, a statistic that alarmed and angered me.

2011

Another Lost Year

"If you could escape from your sufferings, and did so, where would you go outside them?"
— ANTONIO PORCHIA

By spring of 2011, more uncomfortable symptoms arose – a new brand of anxiety, bouts of vertigo, tremors, off-and-on memory lapses, gastrointestinal issues and a pervasive flu – became my 24-hour-a-day companions.

I did not – yet – know that I was developing a 'tolerance'. I only knew that my body was begging me to take more, which I refused to do.

An internal force kept driving me to end my Ativan nightmare. I knew I had to release my body and brain from the insidious effects of the Ativan, as well as the additional sleeping pills my primary doctor prescribed.

My psychiatrist continued to dismiss Professor Ashton's recommendation to undergo a gradual tapering off, buffered by Valium.

The worst part was that two qualified physicians, one psychiatrist, and one addiction specialist, advised that I could keep taking Ativan for the rest of my life, because I was "old," 72 at the time. So I continued on the path put forth by my trusted physicians.

That was just one of the errors I made while trying to understand what had happened to my brain – not my mind, as was the consensus of many practitioners I consulted. The harshest discovery was that even the doctors did not know what was ahead of me.

Vessel of Ashes

My brain is seeping

out of my head.

Flash framed bizarre

images.

Panic

I do not know how

to get out of this

pinhole of a life.

No, not a life.

A gray, numb

existence.

Like a grave.

Like a vessel of ashes.

Enough!

Sunday, December 4, 2011, evening...

Swallow, Spit, Soul
I do not know how to live
I do not know how to die
I exist
A lie
a shape
a shell
a broken heart – mind – psyche – spirit
So now I swallow herbs instead of drugs
and I shake, grit my teeth, swallow, spit
Anxiety creeps in like lava...ooze takes over my soul.
Do I have a soul? I used to be so sure
And now? no surety
just glimmers
I hope once I leave this world, body, mind
I will understand, why, this happened

Part **II**

January, 2012

Bottoming Out, Getting Out

"Near me nothing but distances."
— ANTONIO PORCHIA

In early November while watching the Dr. Murray/Michael Jackson criminal trial, in came Dr. W, a Lorazepam (Ativan/Valuim) expert witness from a celebrity-friendly treatment center in Southern California. Frustrated after several months tapering the Ativan, shaving tiny slivers off each pill, having decreased my dosage by more than half. I called the owner of the facility who told me they could get me off the rest of the Ativan.

With that goal, on January 1 I entered their 30-day residential treatment program.

During my month-long self-incarceration, two doctors, the one I saw on TV and a consulting psychiatrist, rapidly detoxed me of the remaining Ativan in two weeks, using other pills delivered in little white cups, three times a day.

This rather archaic approach to benzodiazepine withdrawal set me up for the Protracted Withdrawal Syndrome, or PAWS, Professor Ashton talks about in her *Ashton Manual*. I was unaware that 15 to 20 percent of people who get off a benzo too rapidly can develop this debilitating condition.

During that month, ensconced in a private suite, in a lovely white house, overlooking the Pacific Ocean, I was constantly told – actually bullied – by fellow residents and staff that "...all addictions are the same...," that benzo dependence was no different. I was urine-tested every few days and had to attend AA meetings, or I would not be allowed to go to the Sunday evening movie with my rehab companions, who included a dozen honest-to-God addicted souls, from a Southern California socialite alcoholic to a bunch of rich kids with a drug history from pre-teen years.

Sitting in those AA meetings listening to introductions, "my name is ... I am an alcoholic" or "I am an addict" when my turn came around I said "My name is Marjorie and I am here to get off benzos" it was clear they did not know what I meant.

I tried to share with the staff what I had learned about benzodiazepines being a very different demon than alcohol, cocaine and other psychoactive drugs – to no avail. The consensus was, even from the therapist to whom I was assigned, that I was in denial.

The reality was "they" did not believe me.

When my 30 days ended, the doctors suggested that I stay longer, even though my mission to rid my system of the remaining Ativan was accomplished.

I declined. So they sent me home with prescriptions for Neurontin and Seroquel, as well as a recommendation to see a psychiatrist.

I declined their prescriptions.

I returned to Oregon Ativan-free, as Dr. W had promised. I thought I had beaten the rap.

Wednesday, February 1, 2012, afternoon...

Home
I am home.
Snow on the ground,
crisp cold air in my lungs.
I walk in the front door
almost cheerful.
I did it, I think.
I made it through,
I am fine
really I am fine.

The discombobulation began two weeks later, as intense withdrawal-like symptoms came on with a vengeance. I was in the purgatory of PAWS.

PAWS (Post Acute Withdrawal Syndrome or Protracted Withdrawal Syndrome)

In simple terms, benzodiazepines work to suppress activity and communication between nerves and neurotransmitters. Prolonged use of a benzo essentially rewires the way the nerves communicate with each other.

When a patient stops taking the benzodiazepine, the brain has to relearn how to communicate with the nerves. This is an extremely slow process and the patient can suffer from horrible side effects while the brain reconnects with the nervous system. The amount of time required for healing can take months or in some cases years to recover.

Sunday, March 11, 2012, morning...

Happy Birthday Milton Carmen
Here I sit on a beautiful spring morning, shaking so badly that it is hard to keep my fingers on the computer keyboard, or focus on the words that are lining up on the screen. I have not slept for more than two hours in the last forty-eight. My brain feels like a bowling ball and it is hard to keep my head from falling forward. Even my saliva gags me. I won't write about my bowels. That is beyond ridiculous. The hissing in my ears does not stop unless I put earphones on and listen to Chopin. The thought of food disgusts me. I cannot go anywhere.

Desperate for any hint of a way out of this abyss, I took heart from advice by Robert Whitaker, author of *Mad In America, Bad Science, Bad Medicine, and the Enduring Mistreatment of the Mentally Ill*:

"Withdrawal does not last indefinitely. Recovery is imminent; it is just a matter of time, patience, hope and courage. So, although the word 'healing' is used frequently, just remember that withdrawal syndrome is not an illness; ...a syndrome is a cluster of symptoms that occur at the same time.

"In the case of benzodiazepines, the nervous system is in a temporary state of being excessively excitable and overly sensitive to stimuli. When the recovery process is complete, the symptoms will subside, you will exhale, celebrate and then enjoy doing everything you couldn't do while you waited for the bumpy ride to end.

"The most important thing to keep in mind is that as unpleasant and unsettling as it can be for many, withdrawal does not last indefinitely. Thousands before you have survived this and are now enjoying fully functional lives once more. This too, will pass..."[10]

Friday, May 4, 2012, morning...

Befuddled

Totally befuddled again this morning. Needing to quiet my mind and body, I listen to yet another teaching from one of the early meditation gurus: Goldstein, Kornfield, Kabat-Zinn, Adyashanti.[11]

They counsel: Still the mind, still the heart, breathe in.

Fill the lungs. Hold. Breathe out. A deep cleansing breath.

This is basic meditation, I realize. But I need basics, back to a square one recovery process. I need to put one foot ahead, then another – one day at a time.

I sink under, with the reality of how my body actually feels. The utter exhaustion that I have to push through each day, continuing gastro-intestinal issues, even after the two-plus months avoiding gluten and dairy.

Absolutely no appetite.

It may be easy to classify me as a 73-year-old depressed, stubborn, lazy, fear-filled woman who just won't get off her ass and find a new purpose for living.

When in fact, I am striving everyday to get out of bed and find purpose in being alive.

A Prayer
May I dwell in my heart
May I be free from suffering
May I be at Peace
May I be healed and whole
Breathe in...hold...breathe out...
— COMMON BUDDHIST CHANT

Tuesday, June 12, 2012, evening...

Reflections on My Self-Incarceration
Six months after returning from that plush celebrity rehab setting, I was not cured.

I had not "beaten the rap" I was lost, again, still.

I kept hauling myself to doctors and practitioners of every sort – internists, acupuncturists, Reiki, neuro-feedback – trying to find something to offset the escalated anxiety, insomnia, sour-tasting nausea, hissing in my ears, quivering, hypersensitivity to light and sound, and more.

When I called Dr. W., the Lorazepam expert, he rudely informed me that "...in the twenty years I've been getting people off these things, I have never had a patient having withdrawal symptoms this far out. No, you need to see a psychiatrist and get on an anti-depressant."

Sixty-thousand dollars later, I realized there was no place for a benzo-dependent person to go to recover. A hard lesson learned.

Now what to do about it?

Wednesday, July 4, 2012, morning...

Tsunami
The Tsunami
My mornings begin in the middle of the night.
I am jolted awake after maybe two hours of a restless sleep.
Then, the tsunami crawls up from my toes and into my gut.
There, it swirls around.
Followed by dry gagging if I even think about food.
What if I am actually losing my mind?
What if this horrific anxiety is eating my neurons?
What if I cannot find my way back to a real life?

These are the questions that pummel me as I sit and tap out random letters, one by one, while my body is a muddle of confusion, having had so little sleep for so many months.

I am living in the fear column, unable to shift my thinking.

What happened to me? What is happening to me?

Is this what is meant by having a "nervous breakdown?"

So, tomorrow I will have a CAT scan of my abdomen and pelvis to see if there is something organic going on that has been causing all these symptoms. I am convinced it must be cancer.

The real issue is: do I want to live enough to go through whatever is to come?

Tuesday, August 7, 2012, 6:00 a.m...

Blink
I stare at the large rectangular computer monitor, blinking
dry eyes, wishing away the tight forearms, hands, listening to
my heart pound in my chest. A panic attack?
I will myself to relax, knowing it too shall pass. It always does.
At six this morning, after maybe three hours of restless
sleep, I awakened with an electric-like jolt, knowing that
another day was outside my bedroom window, yet with no

impetus to do anything in it. I forced myself to eat a remnant from last night's dinner, washed my face, stared at the woman in the mirror like the stranger I was becoming to myself.

So, is this what I am supposed to do? Reveal the persistent agony for any and all to witness? So unlike me, or the me who used to be. The me who hears a quote in my ear, paraphrasing Antonio Porchia, that I remember as:

"Only when you see everything empty itself will you know how to fill it."

Is this the blessing of withdrawal? The emptiness? Is it through this vulnerability that peace will find its way back into my mind and heart? Did I really have to plunge into this valley of the benzo shadows to find a link to a new life?

Help!

Seven months benzo free, I began writing to people and organizations I kept finding online, hoping someone would help me find a protocol that would address this debilitating condition.

Dear (Benzo Contact),

I am writing to enlist your help in bringing attention to a widespread worldwide epidemic: the misuse and overuse of benzodiazepines, as well as other bio-psychiatric drugs that have blunted the brains of millions for decades.

Much of the blame for this travesty must be traced to the giant psychopharma industry, whose primary motivation is profit.

Secondly, most of our trusted physicians are not properly informed as to the dangers of "accidental addiction" and a Post-Acute Withdrawal Syndrome (PAWS) when a patient tries to get off these prescribed, not abused, medications.

Another sad reality is that medical schools do not as yet spend nearly enough time educating our future physicians regarding nutrition, as well as the myriad of side effects that can occur to every organ of the body.

All one needs to do is Google "benzodiazepines" to begin the search for information that is much more available in the UK, Australia, and New Zealand than in the USA. Here, none of the practitioners I consulted knew what the hell I was talking about when I said it was my brain that was messed up, not my mind.

I would appreciate your help in alerting your contacts, both personal and professional, to the dangers, impact of, and solutions to this epidemic.

Sincerely,
Marjorie Carmen

No one responded.

Friday, August 10, 2012, morning...

Un-masked
Third year
memorializing Milton
grieving
finally grieving
The Ativan mask
removed

Tuesday, August 28, 2012, afternoon...

Toxic Sleep
Almost September, while my mind is still sorting out the events of the past six months. On one of the internet's benzo forums, I found the best description of my sleep disorder. The anonymous writer – which is how these groups are run – calls it Toxic Sleep:

"The toxic sleep I experience is a feeling of a kind of half-asleep, accompanied by an overall feeling of irritation and anxiety swirling round and round in my mind. It feels like a

trap, almost like sleep paralysis. We are healing every day we do not swallow any of those evil pills. Amen."

Saturday, August 30, 2012, evening...

A Dead Freezer

Imagine something like discovering a dead freezer at eleven o'clock at night greeting you when all you wanted was some ice cream to soothe a dry, sour mouth. Causing a full-fledged panic attack, I folded to the floor, unable to move. I fell asleep like that, thinking, when I wake I will be strong enough to get up.

Friday, August 31, 2012, evening...

As overly dramatic as this may seem, while Louisiana and other Southern states are wading through the aftermath of Hurricane Isaac, since last night a tsunami-like benzo wave has incapacitated me. Unless it has to do with the Blue Moon I keep hearing about. Whatever it is or is not, my brain/body/ chest/belly/legs/arms/feet feel they are under attack.

Physician: Do No Harm

Still trying to find the antidote to the Ativan poisoning to which I had been subjected for four years, I took all my miserable symptoms to my primary care physician. I had previously given him Heather Ashton's piece on Post Acute Withdrawal Syndrome (PAWS) as well as Baylissa Frederick's message to physicians.[12] He did not believe that, after nine months off Ativan and Trazadone, I could still be coping with benzo withdrawal.

Other than ordering a battery of blood tests, his advice? An anti-depressant. Celexa? Zoloft?

"I don't feel depressed," I told him. Empty, yes. Sad, definitely. Still grieving Milton's death. I finally understand that the Ativan masked the grief I am now experiencing three years later.

Saturday, September 15, 2012, morning...
Family Ties

At 8:30 in the morning, while I was hovering over the toilet, throwing up the oatmeal I was told to eat to heal my gut, the phone rang. By the time I crawled back to the bedroom and answered, I heard my daughter's haranguing voice, chastising me for "being so negative all the time/wasting my life/not inviting the family over for dinner/never being happy"...and on and on.

I had no rebuttal, it was true, but why didn't she care?

I told her if I wanted to fake an illness, I would have chosen an ailment people believed actually existed, or at least believed what I was going through. "Your doctor said you are a hypochondriac," she spit back.

"Benzo-itis does not look as it feels," I replied.

My son, on the other hand, simply ignored me completely. It took a while to realize that those closest to me were the furthermost away.

Then I remembered something from my sojourn at the Graduate Theological Union in Berkeley, California. There, in the early 1990s, I studied God like some people study the stock market.

According to Mark 3:21, when Jesus left home to begin his ministry, members of his family disapproved. "Out of his mind," they said, and some of them attempted to "take charge of him" and bring him home.

Matthew 12:46-50 indicates that he refused to talk to his mother and brothers when they tracked him down. John 7:5 says, "Even his own brothers did not believe in him."

I am learning, those who work together to fulfill the Will of God are the true family, regardless of any blood kinship they might accidentally share.

Monday, October 1, 2012, afternoon...
Pinpricks

Remember that kid Pig Pen in the Peanuts comics? The one who was always engulfed in his own unwashed cloud? I am about to become his crazy aunt.

Vanity forces me to shower, the water becomes pinpricks, makes me want to scream. I must wash away the negative dust in my benzodized brain, focus on this new solo life as it is, not as it was, or how desperate I am for this post-benzo nightmare to end.

Applesauce

I live in what is called a resort retirement community, which translates to a complex of apartments, assisted living quarters and a memory care facility, all situated on beautifully maintained grounds. All is not so beautiful for the residents living with the various indignities and diseases of advancing age.

Case in point: this morning, a man who lives in my building shot himself in the head. This is the first time I fully understand how someone would choose that exit over living in agony.

Have I reached that pinnacle? Am I ready to jump ship? My version would be Seconal, Nembutol, and to make the concoction palatable, applesauce.

So, if I say this to a therapist, I will be deemed depressed and offered yet another pharma cocktail. Best to keep quiet about it, and if it gets too tempting, just Do It! The statistics on benzo-related suicides and murders are troubling.[13]

"Our journey through the dreck and dross of our messes
is an invitation to an enlargement of the soul. Some of these
messes will be our great teachers, some will cause us to grow,

*and some will bring the fullness of failure to bear on the en-
counter with the mystery. Great meaning will often come from
such dismal moments."*
   – James Hollis, Ph.D.[14]

I am still searching for that great meaning.

Early Warnings Unheeded

I discovered Professor Malcolm Lader, a leading expert on the
use and effects of benzodiazepines.[15]
   The following is extracted from an October 6, 2012 letter pub-
lished in *The Times* (UK) from Professor Malcolm Lader.[16]

   *"Sir, I welcome the careful reporting of the use of the ben-
zodiazepine tranquilizers. This controversy has grumbled on
since the first alarms were raised by my research team among
others, in the 1970s. Official warnings have been largely ig-
nored by the prescribers. Two approaches are needed.*
   *"First, the prescription of benzodiazepines should be totally
discouraged. Second, specialized clinics should be expanded
countrywide, not curtailed.*
   *"Requiring these clinics to treat the entire range of sub-
stance abuse problems is totally inappropriate and even coun-
terproductive as my patients used to insist.*
   *"...Long-term usage is being deemed by GP experts in med-
ico-legal cases as possible substandard care, so personal injury
law will come to govern these prescribing practices."*

   *– Malcolm Lader, OBE, LLB, DSc, PhD. FRC
   PSYCH, FMedSci. Emeritus Professor of Clinical
   Psychopharmacology, King's College London.*

   (Used with Malcolm Lader's permission.)

From: meretcarmen
Sent: 10 November 2012 01:01
To: Lader, Malcolm
Subject: Seeking your help

Greetings Professor Lader,
I have been reading many of your articles about the horrors
of Benzodiazepine dependence, totally amazed that so little
information is available here in the United States.

Very briefly, I am ten months Benzo-Free after a four year
dependency on Ativan (prescribed prior to and after my
husband's demise).

Unfortunately, after months of tapering I took the advice of an
addiction specialist and entered a thirty day treatment center
where I was "rapidly" detoxed from the remaining Ativan.
About a week after returning home I began having an array of
symptoms that now fit into Post/Protracted Acute Withdrawal
Syndrome.

At this juncture, I am in utter agony most of the time... but from
everything I have read, the only "cure" is TIME.

Doctors here just want me to take other psychotropic
medications.

Do you know of any protocol from which I might benefit?

Sincerely,
Marjorie Carmen

He was kind enough to respond:

"...time is the main healer!"

Regards,
Professor Malcolm Lader

This correspondence began an invaluable three year email exchange.

Who has the answer to PAWS?

The subject of PAWS has been haunting me since becoming benzo-free. In early November I began delving into the many categories of neuroscience. On the benzo.org.uk website from the Institute of Neuroscience/New Castle (Professor Ashton's venue) I learned neuroscience is the study of the nervous system – including the brain, the spinal cord, and networks of sensory nerve cells, or neurons, throughout the body. Not just from the neck up.

I learned humans contain roughly 100 billion neurons. These are the functional units of the nervous system. They communicate with each other by sending electrical signals long distances and then release chemicals called neurotransmitters which cross synapses – small gaps between neurons.

The nervous system consists of two main parts. The central nervous system, made up of the brain and spinal cord; and the peripheral nervous system, which includes the nerves that serve the neck and arms, trunk, legs, skeletal muscles, and internal organs. This is known as the enteric nervous system, or our "second brain." It is what some call the brain-gut connection.

Apparently, this mass of neural tissue, filled with neurotransmitters, does much more than merely handle digestion or inflict the occasional nervous pang. The little brain in our innards, in connection with the big one in our skulls, partly determines our mental state and plays key roles in certain diseases throughout the body.

"The second brain doesn't help with the great thought processes... religion, philosophy and poetry is left to the brain in the head," says Michael Gershon, chairman of the Department of Anatomy and Cell Biology at New York–Presbyterian Hospital/Columbia University Medical Center, an expert in the nascent field of neurogastroenterology and author of the 1998 book *The Second Brain*.[17]

So I still question which discipline should be responsible for solving PAWS – tweaks to the nervous system or psychiatric treatment? Or both?

Please

Night falls softly

on the discontented

Another day slogged through

disconnected

waiting

for something

anything

Grace...Mercy...Peace

at least

sleep

Please,

sleep

Monday, November 26, 2012, evening...

Wallowing and Whining

That is exactly what it feels like I am doing – wallowing and whining in misery, horribly embarrassed that I have spiraled down so far, trying to understand how this has happened.

Today I saw my primary care physician – the one who ran all those blood tests, GI series, etc.

"All normal," he reports.

"Then why am I so sick?" I asked.

Condescendingly, he explained that psychological factors can cause physiological symptoms. Reading so much as I have about the benzos could result in...in... OK, I thought, he does think I am a hypochondriac.

Then he suggested that I take an anti-depressant for a while to see if that would calm down some of the symptoms I was attributing to PAWS, but that I would have to commit to several weeks of getting adjusted to it. I began to sweat.

So that is where I am right now. What more do we know beyond the right now?

I keep dragging out *The Ashton Manual/2011 supplement*, especially the section on PAWS, and a list of my ongoing symptoms to one doctor or alternative practitioner after another.

I ask them to Google PAWS, Heather Ashton, Malcolm Lader, to get an idea of what I am going through. They stare back at me as if I am speaking Greek.

It seems many people knew that benzodiazepines could ultimately cause brain damage, but not the medical practitioners I've consulted. It is all here in these books I've been asking Amazon to send me. Now it's also here in mine.

Protracted Benzodiazepine (Recovery) Syndrome Symptoms

Benzodiazepine withdrawal presents a wide variety of ongoing symptoms. Because everyone reacts differently and healing is non-linear there is no way to predict how long they may last, or in some cases, if they will every go away. I choose to insert (Recovery) to off-set the fear factor and to remind people that most of us do heal.

Following is a list of symptoms I have endured since weaning myself from the Ativan in January 2012. Some lessen then return; some are made worse by stress or other triggers, or may arise at unexpected times, and for no apparent reason. They may last for a short while or longer. I was told by more than one physician that I had an underlying anxiety disorder.

- Anxiety/panic attacks
- Tremors
- Tinnitus – almost constant; an electrical current.... sometimes louder than others
- Insomnia – 2–3 hours of restless sleep, sometimes less.
- Headaches – shooting pains, brain shivers, brain fog
- Tightness in hands and arms – Paresthesia
- Constant flu symptoms
- Unusual fatigue, weakness, nausea
- Sweating – triggered by fear, negative thoughts, real problems
- Pain in neck and shoulders
- No appetite
- Hair shedding
- Restless legs
- Depersonalization – detached; like being an onlooker of my life
- Derealization – looking through a veil; a sensory fog
- Hallucinations – flashes of visual scenes
- Muscle pain and stiffness
- Vertigo
- Delirium – mostly in the morning after so little sleep
- Anhedonia – unable to feel pleasure
- Muscle spasms

- Intrusive thoughts and memories
- Morbid thoughts
- Agoraphobia
- Gastrointestinal problems – diarrhea or constipation
- Hypersensitivity: light, sound, smell

Monday, December 24, 2012, afternoon...

Masking Grief

Negativity consumes me. I know the tools of the trade: the power of positive affirmations, the value of consistent exercise, good nutrition, therapy, the miracles of prayer.

Nothing connects.

What if all this misery is not the remnants of the GABA deregulation I have read about?

What if all this misery is delayed grief, as the latest of my therapists suggests?

What if, after caring for my husband for so long, masking that grief with Ativan for two years before and two years after he died, is what this agony is all about?

Maybe I need to stop bleeding all over these pages.

GABA (gamma-aminobutyric acid) is a chemical messenger that is widely distributed in the brain. Its natural function is to reduce the activity of the neurons to which it binds. Researchers believe that one of the purposes that GABA[18] serves is to control the fear or anxiety experienced when neurons are overexcited.

2013

Living Benzo-free, Year Two

"I have come one step away from everything. And here I stay, far from everything, one step away."
— ANTONIO PORCHIA

In 1992, I spent a month in Israel with a University of California-Berkeley archaeological team digging up the Biblically noted city of Bethsaida. It was a month of riding in buses with armed soldiers and toiling in the hot summer sun in dust and dirt.

I was thrilled when, after carefully brushing the dust off a small mound, I discovered the rim of a first-century bowl, according to the dig's Israeli director. He explained how you can tell the entire story of a civilization from such a shard.

Similarly, digging into this benzo blunder, and trying to get to the bottom of what happened to me, feels equally daunting. It is a journey I feel compelled to share with the millions of benzo-afflicted people I am finding all over the world.

For instance, a March, 1988 piece by Dr. RF (Reg) Peart, BSc, PhD., cites Professor Malcolm Lader calling benzodiazepines "the Opium of the Masses."[19] And in 1981, Dr. Peart warned of an "epidemic in the making." In 1998, he also stated that benzodiazepine dependence was the largest iatrogenic (medically induced) epidemic of the 1980s.

I am getting very pissed off that none of that information wafted over from England and into the hands of the doctors who pushed me into this benzo hell.

"May I dwell in the heart
"May I be free from suffering
May I be healed
May I be at peace." [20]
— COMMON BUDDHIST PRAYER

I listen to more meditations from Jack Kornfield, Steven Gray (aka Adyashanti), Kabat-Zinn, all telling me that I am not my thoughts, not my feelings, not my personality. That I am more than meets the eye, ear, brain, body. Yet I feel so much less – a nothing.
What will it take to convince me that the past is nothing?
That the future is nothing?
That all I have is this moment...
So what if I do not like it?
So what if I just endure, existing until my body becomes dead flesh and charred bones?
So what if "this is all there is? " (à la singer Peggy Lee)
Is the all enough?
Is that the gist of it, Lord?

Sunday, March 31, 2013, morning...

Another Easter
Still the agony
No ecstasy
No resurrection
Just this miserable anxiety
Stiff arms
greet me each morning

Wednesday, April 10, 2013, evening...

Dark Night of the Soul

*April, and Dark nights continue to plague me as I strive
to endure this benzo-dized existence. Is there a point to this
suffering?*

According to Marla Estes, author of *Making the Unconscious
Conscious: Embracing the Dark Night of the Soul,*[21] *"one of the
symptoms of the dark night of the soul is no longer having any sense
of solid ground."*

One of her definitions of enlightenment is to make the uncon-
scious, conscious. Dark nights are one way to get there.

Marla quotes Marion Woodman, a Jungian analyst:

> *"Creative suffering burns clean; neurotic suffering creates
> more soot."*

Marla continues *"There is a big difference between wallowing
in non-productive and repetitive pain and using the opportunity
of these deep and powerful emotions to bring greater self-under-
standing and ultimately greater liberation from our stuckness and
repetitive patterns."*

My suffering, I believe, has been neurotic.

Thank You, Joseph Campbell

Eighteen months into this benzo-free existence, I am still
searching for physical and psychological solid ground. I find com-
fort in turning to Joseph Campbell, *A Joseph Campbell Companion:
Reflections on the Art of Living:*[22]

> *"Whatever your fate is, whatever the hell happens, you
> say, 'This is what I need.' It may look like a wreck, but go at it
> as though it were an opportunity, a challenge. If you bring*

*love to that moment – not discouragement – you will find
the strength is there. Any disaster that you can survive is an
improvement in your character, your stature, and your life.
What a privilege! This is when the spontaneity of your own
nature will have a chance to flow. Then, when looking back at
your life, you will see that the moments which seemed to be
great failures followed by wreckage were the incidents that
shaped the life you have now. You'll see that this is really true.
Nothing can happen to you that is not positive. Even though
it looks and feels at the moment like a negative crisis, it is
not. The crisis throws you back, and when you are required to
exhibit strength, it comes."*

Saturday, June 1, 2013, afternoon...

Is it PAWS?

*Constant Flu. From the moment I open my eyes and
throughout the day, choking at the mere thought of food.*

Even food ads on TV make me gag.

*From what I glean from all the Googling I do in the middle
of the night, looking up things such as "the brain on benzos," it
looks as if my appetite center, along with my sleep center, both
apparently located in the hypothalamus area in the brain,
have been zapped by the affair with Ativan.*

*From what I gather from Heather Ashton, I believe I am one
of the elite 15-20 percent of former benzo-dependent patients
who have become PAWS sufferers, most likely due to the rapid
detox I chose to do last year. As yet, there are no protocols to
assist people to full benzo recovery. I intend to find them and
to share them.*

Thursday, June 20, 2013, afternoon...

Echoes of Ativan

Today I am coping with the constant hissing/
electromagnetic tinnitus, just one of the protracted
annoyances. There is no rhyme or reason for this non-linear
healing process; no way of predicting what symptoms are
going to pop up when or where.

I have learned to expect this uncertainty, given what
I am reading about the up- and down-regulated GABA[23]
receptors. I read stories about people like me, who,
decades later, are still struggling with these echoes
of Ativan.

Friday, June 28, 2013, afternoon...

Words

So many words, from so many self-help gurus, all saying the
same thing. You are not your thoughts and ideas. You are mere
awareness, nothing more or less. Be the witness of what goes
on inside of you. Change happens by itself. Act from that state
of pure awareness. Awareness does not create suffering.

Awareness is not needy. Acting out of the egoic mind (a
state of mind in which the ego is in control of your thoughts
and emotions), you make the present moment a means to an
end. Action out of selflessness. Zen, no self, no problem. Live
and act with a mentally constructed self. Don't personalize it.

But this does feel intensely personal.

Mindfulness

Last April, I took an eight-week Mindfulness Stress Reduction
Seminar, led by Ray Gertler, Ph.D. There, I was introduced to formal
and informal Awareness techniques as a way to calm my hyper-
sensitive nervous system. Like meditation in general, but without

a totally Buddhist perspective, this practice is a discipline that has to be cultivated over time.

As I noted in my class journal, from an unknown source, "Like a flood lamp instead of a spotlight, mindfulness illuminates a more fluid field of ever-changing experiences, rather than isolating a particular object for intensive scrutiny. This alternative mode of observation is necessary because mindfulness practice is more about investigating a process than about examining an object."

I have not been successful in setting aside a disciplined mindfulness practice, which is encouraged by teachers like Jon Kabat Zinn and Pema Chodron. But I have learned breathing techniques that stave off the panic that comes with benzo withdrawal. And I do understand that the intention is to tap into a greater awareness – moment by moment.

Monday, July 29, 2013, afternoon...

The Practice

How easy it is to let go of the discipline needed to make meditation a priority in my life. I am least likely to try it when I most need it – on awakening, usually in the middle of the night. I am immediately plunged into a cacophony of life skits playing across my mind. I sit in a room with six television sets, all on different channels, talking heads in competition with each other. I am pulled into decisions I'm not clear about yet. The novel I was/am hoping to complete looks ridiculous. Perhaps my back may be in jeopardy.

Inhale, focus, exhale. Inhale, focus, exhale. Make space around the rhythm of the breath. When one skit wanders in, acknowledge its presence and place it in the realm beyond reason, or whatever you call the trusted but unseen energies some call the God name. Like that which I cannot change, it is a challenge to change my relationship to it.

Saturday, August 10, 2013, evening...

Romancing the Clock
Chimes
the tick tock
time, reminders
of four years past
a day that is
as if tomorrow

Tuesday, August 20, 2013, afternoon...

I lay prostrate on the living room floor, my forehead pressed into the neglected, dusty carpet, arms stretched out like a cross. I called on my academic theological education, Christian and otherwise, Kabbalistic mysticism, with some Buddhist-like wisdom tossed into the mix.

I cried out from the depth of my pain, "Hear my prayer... take me Home..."

At that point, John Denver wafted in singing the next line, "country road." I started laughing, remembering something a Buddhist monk once told me. He stood before me in his orange robe, a knowing smile on his shining face. "Aren't you taking life a little too seriously, Marjorie?"

Smiling to myself, I got up.

Squirming
I awoke at 3:00 a.m. again, bathed in a cold sweat.
Another wave-tossed night.
Broken sleep.
Now, several hours later, I just sit.

Saturday, September 14, 2013, morning...

The view – which should calm me – is over evergreens piercing a powder blue cloudless sky.

Another panic attack!

Several this week, a normal part of healing those blunted GABA receptors, according to what I've read.

Maybe I am going off that deep end I hear so often attributed to someone who "lost it," like in the 1976 film *Network*. I recall the infamous scene in which Howard Beale (Peter Finch) tells the people:

> *"I don't want you to protest. I don't want you to riot. I don't want you to write to your congressman... First you've got to get mad. You've got to say I'm a human being, God damn it! My life has value! So I want you to get up now. I want all of you to get up out of your chairs. I want you to get up right now and go to the window. Open it and stick your head out, and yell:* **"I am mad as hell and I am not going to take this anymore!"**

So who dropped the benzo ball in the U.S? Where were the warnings about benzos? So yes, I am mad. As in angry, as in crazy. So what!

Pharma's Great Wrath

Surging

I awaken to a silent house

No demands from anyone

Perceptual sounds are electronic

Wires, wireless, waves, particles

Surging around invisibly

Penetrating my compromised

Nervous systems

Still healing from

Pharma's Great Wrath

Monday, October 31, 2013, afternoon...

What Happens?
On the way home from yet another doctor appointment I almost ran my car off the Bill Healy Bridge.

Finished
What happens when you are hanging
on to faith, hope, God, and trust
even if you do not feel any of it?
Who just gives up,
buys a gun
shoots herself
on All Hallows Eve?
Would I?
Could I?
find a less bloody way
like in applesauce
To go Home?
Would I choose to "end it"
Now
if I could?
before I finish
This Story I Came To Tell
(truth be told, yes.)

Saturday, December 14, 2013, afternoon
Cyber Universe

Feeling I may actually expire before I make it out of this Benzo-itis, I contacted an IT consultant to help me enter the cyber universe. With his help I created an educational forum called Advocates for Social Reform.

I did not know at the time I would use this platform for much more than to complete the writing I have been doing for more than fifty years, some published, most not.

Christmas Eve in Purgatory

The word "Purgatory" is derived from the Latin purgatorium and refers to a wide range of historical and modern concepts of temporary postmortem suffering or torment.[24]

According to Roman Catholic teaching, the theological notion of Purgatory is a temporary state of purification. In Eastern churches it is called a Final Purificatrion or Theosis (coming to a Union with God). John Wesley, who founded Methodism, believed in an intermediate state between death and the Final Judgment.

An excellent metaphor for A Protracted Benzodiazepine (Recovery) Syndrome, especially on Christmas Eve.

2014

Little Did I Know

"I hold up what I know with what I do not know."
— ANTONIO PORCHIA

I entered my third year free from all psychoactive pharmaceuticals, alternative medicinal combinations and other plant based products, yet still in a protracted misery that comes and goes under its own volition.

My journey through the benzo miasma has been marked by milestones of discovery: the "little did I know" moments. Had I been armed and informed with the information herein, I might have avoided my agonizing descent and slow, painful recovery of my brain and body's withdrawal from benzodiazepines.

Wednesday, January 1, 2014, morning...

Power Outage
I look out at a frozen forest
icy snow crystals floating down
coating the Ponderosas
like powdered sugar
on Christmas tree cookies
I am powerless
caught in a wave of benzo anxiety

Wednesday, January 8, 2014, afternoon...

If Wishes Were Horses, Then Beggars Would Ride

I continually doubt the impact of sharing my journey through benzo hell. How I wish I felt more confident, that by excavating my own prolonged benzo dilemma, and "living sick," as I have for the last two years, my story will at least make a dent in the armored fortress of the bio-pharmaceutical industry.

Friday, February 14, 2014
Bad Pharma

On a plane to Florida to visit my daughter and son in-law, who still thought of me as "malingering." I spent the hours wading through Ben Goldacre's *Bad Pharma*,[25] horrified by what I read about pharmaceutical deceit and avarice.

Meanwhile, I continue my mission to shed new light on an old subject – the benzo-dization of our culture. The material I have dredged up over the last two-plus years is overwhelming. How can it have a positive impact on a system so shattered, first by ignorance and then by greed?

So here I am, twenty-six months benzo-free, still quaking with flu-like symptoms. I've lived through twenty-six months of chronic insomnia, no appetite whatsoever, and the electronic hissing from tinnitus; still "living sick."

I know there are thousands like me, including:

- those realizing that the pills they have been swallowing no longer quell their anxiety.
- those trying to taper off.
- those who, like me, have become one of the protracted, plagued with an even higher degree of neuro/physio/psycho symptoms than when they first sought help.

None of this would have happened had Malcolm Lader and Heather Ashton's pleas for further research been heeded decades ago.

There must be some justice in all of this – some accountability.

Maybe I have to stage a hypothetical class action suit to, find one CEO of one pharmaceutical corporation, to see the value of acknowledging something that must be corrected for the sake of new generations.

Yes, I know. Fat chance.

Tuesday, March 11, 2014, afternoon...

Happy 90th Birthday, Milton Carmen

"How do I live when you're not here? Pain lives me, a wound speaks with my mouth. And when you return?

"Only you know how you hollow me out and dance in the hollow." – Jalal-ud-Din Rumi

Green Medicine

Two years med-free, yet still suffering symptoms of PAWS, it became clear that any prescribed or over the counter medication was creating a paradoxical reaction.

Dr. M suggested that medical cannabis might help with the insomnia, nausea, and waves of tsunami-like anxiety. Following his recommendation I began reading about the benefits of medicinal cannabis and decided to explore the Oregon Medical Marijuana Program.

The process led me to what looked like a medical office. I spent the whole day getting qualified, along with about a dozen "patients" who looked far worse than I.

So, after spending about $400, plus a quick exam from the MD at the state-run office, I received my state issued Medical Marijuana card. I bought a strain of "flower" designated for insomnia and pain and a little marble pipe. I went home feeling rather guilty, even though the State of Oregon deems cannabis legal.

I put a raisin size ball in the bowl of the pipe and lit up. Like a light switch, the whirling dervish in my gut stopped whirling, the salivating nausea let up. For a very short while I felt "normal." That is, until the sweet effect of the green medicine (that is what they call it at the state sanctioned clinic) wore off and I sank back into benzo withdrawal tremors for the rest of the night.

But at least I got some relief.

Not Your Daughter's Cannabis

While cannabis is now more accepted as a medicinal comfort, my introduction to "pot" occurred in the 1970s. I found a plastic bag with a small amount of what was obviously not oregano in my teen daughter's underwear drawer. I pilfered it.

Next, I took one of my then-husband's Winston cigarettes and locked myself in the bathroom. In that safe haven, I twisted the tobacco into the toilet, and, using a perfume funnel, filled the hollowed-out cigarette paper with the crumbled leaves, closed the lid, stood on the toilet, lit up, took one, and then another puff, blowing the smoke into the air vent. Then I got down, sprayed the bathroom with a $110 bottle of Chanel No. 5, immediately feeling the effects of the marijuana.

So, instead of ironing my then-husband's Air Force officer's blue shirts, I got on my bike, rode to our suburban man-made lake, and sitting with my back pressed against a blossoming white dogwood tree, spent the rest of the afternoon reading one of Thoreau's 14 journals.

My daughter never asked about the bag, nor did I mention it. Pot may have been easy for my teenage daughter to obtain, but not her mother. It was years before I saw marijuana again.

In 1976, my sister from Berkeley came to help out while I was recovering from a triple back fusion with bone grafts. That was when I discovered that marijuana was better for pain control than the narcotics they were handing me in those white paper cups that were making me throw up.

More years passed. My next marijuana episode was in graduate school during an acrimonious divorce, and having a charming affair with a gorgeous fellow student.

Memories such as these warm my heart on lonely winter nights.

Dopamine

After receiving even short term relief from the Green Medicine, I found I had to partake rather often to keep the benzo symptoms at bay.

I asked the fellow at the dispensary what cannabis does to the brain to have that effect.

"Dopamine," he said. And when it wears off?

"Just take some more, like aspirin," he said nonchalantly.

Not exactly what I had in mind by turning to this plant to help regain my health.

Then I saw CNN programs, "Weed," "Weed 2: Cannabis Madness," and "Weed 3, The Marijuana Revolution," hosted by Sanjay Gupta. One of the episodes mentioned a particularly cultivated strain of cannabis that had an astonishing effect on an epileptic child, reducing her seizures from hundreds to few.

"Ah ha," I actually said aloud, "There it is."

That is when I began looking for a strain that might create a bridge for people who want to be rid of a benzodiazepine or an antidepressant, or those who are already tapering. Or at least a partial panacea for people like me who are benzo-free but continue to struggle with a central nervous system that has been so blunted.

No luck to date.

Friday, April 18, 2014, afternoon...

Floundering

My days flounder between confidence that this shared journey toward benzo recovery is producing something worthwhile, then sinking into a quagmire of fear that nothing I am doing will convince anyone of anything.

Talking to Your Health Care Provider About Cannabis

The first thing you should do is find a qualified physician or other medical practitioner who is enlightened by the wealth of information available about the curative aspects of Cannabis.

Ask questions to determine if medical cannabis might be helpful for you in possibly avoiding other medications.

- Does medicinal cannabis seem like a good option for my problem?
- What do you know about the medicinal cannabis being cultivated today?
- What are the health risks associated with cannabis use?
- Should I smoke it, eat it, or inhale it?
- Where can I find more information on medicinal cannabis?
- Will I be able to perform my everyday duties while using medicinal cannabis?
- Will I be able to use my medicinal cannabis around my children?
- Will cannabis interact with my other medications?

Exploring these issues does not dismiss statistics indicating a growing minority of frequent users can become psychologically or physically addicted.

What would I be doing were I not planted in my studio all day, moving from file to file? It makes me realize, so much of what I plucked from my months of research has already been said about the havoc benzodiazepines can cause; and how it has been ignored or categorically denied for decades.

In the beginning "they" may not have known that sending psychoactive molecules into our brains over a long period of time would cause our natural GABA receptors to shut down. But "they" sure do now!

Now the question is: What the hell to do about it?

Perhaps an event, gathering together the worlds leading benzo experts to help people like me recover in a sustained and planned process.

This came from the exploration into the process of "restorative" justice as my weapon of choice. Not to castigate or litigate – but to educate!

Easter Saturday

In the 1950s, as a Jewish girl growing up in a Christian neighborhood and going to the Presbyterian Church with my girlfriends, I wondered what happened to Jesus after he was so brutally murdered and before his apparent rising on Easter morning. One day, after the Good Friday event, I looked it up in the Church library and read that he just "lay in the tomb."

Many years later, I began seeing the relevance of those gospel stories; as I was forced to surrender to circumstances out of my control, clinging to faith, the dimensions of which I have yet to understand.

Resurrection? When?

The Easter story has become massacred over the eons, at least from the "academic theological" points of view. The story takes you back to the roots of the Messianic legend and the evolving

New Testament. Not the version that sets Christian against Jew for these two-thousand-plus years.

Two attorney friends have warned me about playing David to the Psycho-Pharma Goliaths, suggesting solutions to this benzo blunder could get me into a lot of legal or other trouble.

Do I care? No.

What I do care about is my newborn granddaughter, whom, I pray, is never offered a benzodiazepine if she is nervous about taking a test – something I'm told is standard practice at one of the local high schools.

Thursday, April 24, 2014, afternoon...

The Long Road Through Recovery

Twenty-eight months benzo-free, inch by inch, hardly noticeable progress, except that I seem to be thinking more clearly, more deeply than I have in four years.

I am beginning to see how my current disillusionment about so much I see and hear – in my own family circle as well as in the world at large – is attached to how I perceive my physicality in relation to presence; spirit/soul. A sense of the eternal lets us know we are not alone in the story of our lives, no matter how difficult our moment-to-moment living feels under the cloud of unknowing[26] I remember reading about ages ago. The anonymous treatise asks one to surrender preconceived notions of God to the "unknowingness" as the path to knowing the true nature of God.

Another mindfulness understanding.

Tuesday, April 29, 2014, afternoon...

Encouragement

A quote from Ben Goldberg's book, Bad Pharma, was terribly enlightening.

"When systems fail, the appropriate response is to admit to the problem and to work hard to fix it."

*This is what I have decided to do. This is the encouragement
I need!*
   A turning point in my recovery.

May Day

"May Day" is a term that came into use in the 1920s as a distress
signal for aviators, approximating the French term m'aider, mean-
ing "come help me!" Until quite recently, my childhood recollection
of May Day had been a tall wooden pole with dozens of colorful
ribbons held by tiny hands as we danced around the pole herald-
ing the arrival of Spring.

No longer. Now I squirm through another one of these benzo
waves I learned of through the Benzobuddies website. Now my
body is issuing May Day alerts; a plea for someone to toss me a
benzo-recovery life preserver.

Sunday, June 1, 2014, evening...

My Face on the Sunday Bend Bulletin
   *9:30 tonight I received a call from the front desk that a
woman from Bend wanted to speak to me about the article
Markian Hawryluk wrote in today's paper.*
   *My face is in the Health Section of the Bend Bulletin. I
have become the "Benzo Babe" of Bend, Oregon.[27] Yet, if this
exposure helps one other benzo-dized victim, I am happy to
recount my benzo journey to the public at large.*

That call led to my hosting a small (three member) benzo
discussion, support, and recovery group, until one member moved
away and the other, a business man, became uncomfortable being
associated with the subject.

There are recovery groups throughout the world – alcoholics
have AA, narcotics users have NA – but nothing for a benzo with-
drawal and recovery process. The stigma of perceived "addiction"

prevents many benzo sufferers from coming out of their own darkness when there is no welcoming committee.

Addiction vs. Dependence – Not Synonyms

Both Addiction and Dependence are often used interchangeably with Drug Abuse, big mistake, it turns out.

According to experts in the field, drug addiction is a behavioral syndrome in which the use of a substance dominates one's life and normal constraints are ineffective against the overwhelmingly powerful motivation to obtain and self-administer the drug. Addiction is a persistent compulsive use of a substance known by the user to be harmful.

In contrast, drug dependence refers to a state in which the individual relies on the drug for normal physiological functioning. Dependence is an adaptive state that develops from repeated drug administration, which results in withdrawal upon cessation of drug use.

Friday, August 8, 2014, morning...

Chickens or Eggs?

I am completely stymied today, probably a result of an unnerving conversation with Dr. M When I asked about having an MRI to see if any brain damage was evident, he responded quite condescendingly, "Well, Marjorie, can you see depression on an X-ray?" Nevertheless, last week I submitted my cranium to the MRI behemoth.

Now it is 10:15 a.m., and I sit here waiting to hear what the MRI indicates.

The report? My cerebral cortex is smaller than average for a woman my age. Is it the result of normal aging processes or the benzos?

Then it dawned on me! Among all these doctors, therapies, even the meditation techniques (Change your Mind, Change your Brain), trying to find something to offset the escalated

anxiety, insomnia, constant nausea, hissing in my ears,
quivering, hypersensitivity, the consensus is that my condition
is "mind" driven.

The bottom line? Without the brain we do not have a
mind. Not the other way around. This was a major "aha"
moment for me.

I Have a Mission

As hard as it is to trust, given the non-linear aspect of benzo
recovery, I do believe that I am getting better. The reawakening of
these complicated GABA receptors is so gradual that, along with
my hypothalamus/pituitary axis[28] being reamed, I have come to
understand what the damn Lorazepam/Remeron/Trazadone/
Gabapentin/Seroquel actually did to my brain.

It seems that now my task is to offer not only hope and faith to
others who have been lured into this benzo trap, but also to take
it steps further by sharing the myriad of healing modalities I've
explored.

What Jesus Said About All of This

In the late 1980s, while living in Carmel, California, I
co-wrote and produced a Christmas play (*Miracle By The Sea*)
with Carol Anstey Richmond. While creating this three-act
musical script, using whatever story we could glean from the
minimal details in the Bible, I became acquainted with the
"historical" Jesus.

This led me to Berkeley's Pacific School of Religion for a year
of studying God, like some study the stock market, taking into
account history, context, evidence, and imagination.

During one of the New Testament courses, I was introduced to
The Gospel of Thomas. Discovered in the 20th century in Coptic[29]
form, and thought by some to have been compiled before the final
four, the gospel (meaning good news) is made up of 114 sayings
attributed to "the Living Jesus."

Number five particularly resonated with me, and in many ways has become one of my personal mantras.

Jesus said, "Know what is in front of your face, and what is hidden from you will be disclosed ...For there is nothing hidden that will not be revealed..."

The Times, They are a'changin...

"Those who do not have power over the story that dominates their lives, the power to retry, rethink it, deconstruct it, joke about it, and change it as times change, truly are powerless"
— SALMAN RUSHDIE

If not anti-anxiety medications and antidepressants, then what? What if nothing offsets traumatic mind and soul jarring events or a persistent depression that will not let up?

Factor in the onslaught of television and magazine ads touting the benefits of one antidepressant after the other – followed by a long list of the risks, including death. Yet, the multitudes flock to their doctors' offices asking for them.

When I asked Dr. M why he still prescribed benzos for his patients, his response was that if he didn't, they would go elsewhere.

"We are a society seeking immediate gratification," he said. "It is our own belief system that drives an imbalance resulting in maladaptive behaviors creating symptoms of anxiety and insomnia.

"Drugs are not always the answer, but the pressure to provide a quick fix is mostly patient-driven, and fueled by advertising campaigns.

"Shouldn't we be asking the hard questions, such as what is driving our anxiety and depression, instead of covering it up with something or anything?"

The good news is that we are not alone in our quest to become psycho-pharma free. "The times, they are a'changin...," as Bob Dylan sang a half-century ago. There is an emerging awareness – unfortunately created by an influx of celebrity overdose headlines – alternatives to pill-popping to help you cope with common life stressors. Luckily, the mantra "you are what you eat" is becoming more widely accepted.

Further, the practice of mindfulness, which teaches us to breathe again, to let go of ego-based clinging, has become more mainstream.

Who Dropped the Benzoball in the USA?

Who should have alerted the US medical community and its patients to the dangers of long-term use of benzos? This is the question that has been plaguing me since discovering the clearly-ignored 525-page transcript of the 1979 Edward Kennedy US Senate subcommittee hearing on the Use and Misuse of Benzodiazepines, infamously became known as the "Valium Hearing."

According to the hearing's transcripts, Valium was routinely taken by 15 percent of the population at that time. The president of Hoffman-La Roche insisted that "the beneficial effects of Valium far outweigh its detrimental effects."

Senator Kennedy responded, "Thousands of Americans are hooked and don't know it."

Kennedy, Food and Drug Administration officials, and doctors concerned about the problem urged a promotional campaign to inform patients and physicians of the dangers. This information was available nearly forty years ago!

Then in 1980, RAUS (Research Analysis and Utilization System) Review Conference on Benzodiazepines/ National Institute on Drug Abuse.[30] The organization's Summary of New Directions for Research by Jacqueline P. Ludford, M.S. and Stephen I. Scara, M.D., D.Sc. noted:

"Future Benzodiazepine research should, first and foremost, be methodologically strong and rigorous. Future investigations need to be based on sound experimental and epidemiological data, and there is much work to be done in developing such data for benzodiazepines. Much of the research already performed has been... flawed and is open to some question."

So, who swept benzos under the rug?

Might it have anything to do with the top twenty pharmaceutical companies and their two trade groups?

Review this checklist, adapted from various websites, whenever a physician prescribes something unfamiliar.

1. How much improvement can I expect, and how soon?
2. If I don't take this drug right now, what will happen?
3. What are the most likely side effects?
4. Are there any rare serious side effects?
5. Are there any permanent problems this drug can cause?
6. Is there an older drug more useful?
7. Can I try a lower dose?
8. When will we review my use of this drug?
9. Are there problems – or any special considerations – to consider when stopping the drug?
10. Are there any potential interactions with food, my other medical conditions, or my current medications?
11. Might this drug affect my weight, sleep, hair, skin, nails, mood, or sex life?

According to the non-partisan Center for Responsive Politics, the Pharmaceutical Research & Manufacturers of America spent almost $20 million on lobbying, just in 2016.

The Center for Public Integrity found that drug companies and allied advocates spent more than $880 million on lobbying and political contributions at the state and federal level over the past decade. Further, the drug companies and allied groups deploy an average of 1,350 lobbyists per year, covering all state capitols.

I think you'll agree, the statistics are staggering!

My dilemma lies in how to contact pharmaceutical companies and get their attention in a non-confrontational way – without having doors slammed in my face.

The U.K. is Far Ahead in Benzo Awareness

The following remarks on October 23, 2013 in the House of Commons, United Kingdom (UK) underscore how far the UK community has come in awareness of the benzo dilemma.

Jim Dobbin, member of Parliament: "A total of 1.5 million people in the UK are addicted to the benzodiazepines, diazepam and 'Z drugs.' I know of one individual who has been on those products for more than 45 years – a total life ruined.

"Will the Prime Minister advise the Department of Health to give some guidance to the clinical commissioning groups to introduce withdrawal programmes in line with the advice from Professor Heather Ashton of Newcastle University, who is the expert in this field, to give these people back their lives?"

David Cameron, Prime Minister: "I join... in paying tribute to Professor Ashton,[31] whom I know has considerable expertise in this area.... These people are not drug addicts, but they have become hooked on repeat prescriptions of tranquilisers. The Minister for Public Health is very happy to... make sure that the relevant guidance can be issued."

Part **III**

2015–2017

Repairing the Benzo Blunder

"When I come upon some idea that is not of this world, I feel as though this world had grown wider."
— ANTONIO PORCHIA

Thursday, January 1, 2015, morning
Time

I can't say it was one of those light bulb "Ah ha!" moments you hear about, but close to it. On the first morning of this year, now three years benzo-free, my eyes opened before the benzo-fueled "ick" began. This repeated morning after morning. Instead of the cortisol rushes that usually shook me awake, something new, Normalcy!

The first thing I thought was something Professor Lader told me three year earlier.

"Time," he said, "is the antidote."

As the weeks sped by more "windows" of normalcy greeted me. The ringing and hissing in my ears diminished, as did the morning choking. I could drink a real cup of Peet's Sumatra coffee, laced with real cream.

The chronic insomnia did not let up. Since sleeping pills were out of the question, I turned to Chinese medicine. I consulted with Holly Hutton, a holistic practitioner, who prescribed tonics and powders to address digestive issues related to the "benzo gut".

I dove into everything I could even remotely understand about the brain and this insidious chemical cocktail Leo Sternbach[32] stirred up, with no idea that there were millions like me. Millions who had the misfortune of discovering what a blind allegiance to an antiquated notion of doctoring did to our brains, and thus, our psyches, bones, and organs.

Gradually, it dawned on me. The story I thought I was writing – my journey through benzo hell and its aftermath, was just the beginning.

As I retraced my steps in and out of Benzoland, waves of all-too-familiar symptoms came back with a vengeance, an uncanny reminder of how vulnerable I was to this non-linear recovery process. All I had to do was think back to the time when the darkest clouds of unknowing enveloped my entire being and the shaking returned.

"I come from dying, not from having been born. From having been born I am going."
— ANTONIO PORCHIA

I Didn't Die. Now What?

"What now?" The woman in the mirror stared back.

"You don't think you are going to make any difference with your little benzo missive, do you?"

The snickering, vindictive voice came from behind me.

Yet the only reflection was mine, albeit a cleaner version than on that harrowing night in 2012, when I was sure I would die before the year was out.

But I didn't die.

2015 became a year when hope took hold. It was a year of many challenges, travel, interviews for this book, and amazing encounters with amazing people. The year I took a quantum leap into the Cyber Universe by starting a blog and a website.

I would say I am mostly recovered. A recovery so arduous I might not have made it through the benzo madness, were it not for an inner fire, fueled by believing my life mattered. A recovery accomplished in spite of the dismissive, condescending attitudes taken by the medical profession and my own family.

Thursday, April 16, 2015
Empathic Therapies

Continuing to seek answers, I registered for Peter Breggin's Empathic Therapy Conference at the Michigan State University Campus. I flew to East Lansing, Michigan for the Conference to learn about healing through Empathic Therapies. I was also introduced to the word "Biopsychiatry" an approach that aims to understand mental disorder in terms of the biological function of the nervous system.

I had the pleasure of meeting Robert Whitaker and hearing him speak. I have been following his work for years.

There are fifteen Guidelines for Empathic Therapy[33] – This one resonated with me the most.

Because human beings thrive when living by their highest ideals, individuals may wish to explore their most important personal values, including spiritual beliefs or religious faith, and to integrate them into their therapy and their personal growth.

Peter Breggin

When I read the information below, from Peter Breggin's book *Your Drug May Be Your Problem, How and Why to Stop Taking Psychiatric Medications*,[34] it felt like a private consultation with someone who understood what I was experiencing.

"When you talk to your doctor about problems stopping or reducing the dose of your psychiatric drug, keep in mind that your doctor may not know much about the problem or may even be irrationally denying its existence. Withdrawal reactions have been repeatedly documented. Yet some doctors seem completely unaware of the existence of these reactions.

"Your doctor may also mistakenly attribute your withdrawal reactions to your 'mental illness.' Especially if you have unsuccessfully tried to withdraw from the drug previously, your doctor may try to convince you that you have a 'chronic illness' requiring lifetime drug use. The irony is that the longer you stay on the drug, the more likely you are to suffer something beyond a mild reaction when you attempt to withdraw. Your unsuspecting doctor, and even you, might see this as a sign that you 'really need' your drug. In reality, what you really need is help in gradually withdrawing."

And he went on...as if I were in his office in New York.

"Withdrawal reactions from benzodiazepines are extremely well documented. Tranquilizers can produce withdrawal reactions often after only a few weeks of use. The longer you take a tranquilizer, the higher the doses, and the more abrupt the withdrawal – the more serious your withdrawal reactions are likely to be. "... Remember that you, and no one else, will do the actual 'work' of coming off drugs. ... You must therefore try to be in charge of the entire process from the very beginning, from the very first moment you decide for yourself that coming off drugs is your goal."

Tuesday, August 25, 2015
The Royal Psychiatrists' International Congress

I returned from a four week journey to the UK as a delegate at the Royal Psychiatrists' International Congress in Birmingham,[35] where I spent three days in the company of over 2,000 psychiatrists from all over the world. There was hardly a mention of Benzodiazepines.

One of the highlights was a daylong meeting with Baylissa Frederick, the founder of Recovery Road and the author of *Recovery & Renewal*. Her "benzo book" helped me understand what the hell was wrong with me during this recovery.

Then on to London, where I finally met Professor Malcom Lader, who kindly read through the first draft of my manuscript.

As recently as a year ago, I would not have had the health or stamina to complete such a journey; a testimony of hope for those still caught in the benzotrap.

You will heal!

"This world understands nothing but words, and you have come into it with almost none."
— ANTONIO PORCHIA

Time to Move On

"Finish the damn thing and get on with it," intoned the voice that started the whole thing.

For weeks, I stared at the manuscript, rereading each fragment from the four year journey, I had inadvertently made through the valley of the shadow of benzo-dependence and its horrifying aftermath.

This is when I saw beyond my own benzo journey and how I might be able to help others through the benzo shadows and into a new life.

"Enough is Sufficient, Sweeney"

That phrase, familiar from childhood, is just one of the literary nicknames my father used (Clytemnestra and Murgatroyd two others) in an attempt to stop my constant "Why-ing" about anything that made me curious.

That same curiosity led me through the belly of the Benzo Beast, where I persevered in spite of alternately wanting to die and to live. Without this drive, or incessant curiosity, I believe I would not have lived to enjoy my present state of recovery.

One story among so many that flood numerous Internet forums, this one about the agony, but ultimately, it is about Recovery.

New Years Eve, December 31, 2015, evening...
**Exaggerated Circumstances Require
Highly Imaginative Solutions**

I cannot think of many more exaggerated circumstances than
the current state of the medical/pharmaceutical industry. At first, I
thought it was just my own stupidity that dumped me into Benzo
Hell. It took more than three years and all the research listed in the
AfterWords of this book to realize that it was not my ignorance,
but that of "qualified" medical practitioners. They were seduced by
an industry that, early on, sacrificed a sacred mandate of Ethical
Responsibility in favor of profit and greed.

So, now what? Sue the bastards?

That has certainly been done, successfully in some cases.

But did we hear about those litigations?

I realized I had accumulated enough evidence, anecdotal in
most cases, to spend the next five years embedded in a lawsuit
against Big Pharma.

For example, did Dr. K, who handed me the first prescription for
Ativan, read any of the articles that could have cautioned her about
prescribing it?

Did we hear about the largest ever class action lawsuit against
drug manufacturers in the UK in the 1980s and 1990s, involving
14,000 patients and 1,800 law firms that alleged the manufactur-
ers knew of the dependence potential but intentionally withheld
this information from doctors?

Did I know, in 2007, when I filled the prescription for Ativan,
that in the UK some doctors were requiring that patients sign a
consent form, indicating they were adequately warned of the risks
before starting treatment with a benzodiazepine?

So where does that bring me on this final morning of 2015,
while I stand in the same bathroom, in front of that same mir-
ror, for a moment reflecting that other woman, the one with the
hollow eyes?

"This world is but a canvas to our imagination"
— HENRY DAVID THOREAU

A Forum for Restorative Justice

One day back in 2014 feeling like a little girl, stamping my feet **"wah wah,** This is **not** fair! This is **not** justice!"

I thought what is justice anyway, so I looked it up.

Ah...here it is: Restorative Justice – Focuses on the needs of victims and offenders, instead of satisfying abstract legal principles or punishing the offender.

Given all the evidence I've unearthed indicating millions of people have been compromised, some permanently, by a long-term relationship with a benzodiazepine. I certainly have a case for a lawsuit. At the very least, I could have my day in court.

It began with an audacious notion, instead of spending a fortune entrenched in the courts, I decided to conduct a New Millennium Social Reform Experiment. Choosing ancient tribal principles, exploring ethical responsibility and a restorative brand of justice, the fragments of what I wanted to do began to fall into place.

Once I discovered Howard Zehr (known as the "grandfather of Restorative Justice"), I began designing a way to apply his work to repairing the benzo blunder using Restorative Practices as my weapons of choice.

It is time for the creators, manufacturers, distributors, and prescribers of benzodiazepines to be called on the carpet and answer to a new jury. Not one in a courtroom with A vs. B.

Learning and Planning

Still dealing with diminished energy, I approached the St. Charles Health System in Bend, Oregon about conducting an International Benzodiazepine Symposium.

After many meetings and discussions, St. Charles signed on to co-sponsor, The International Benzodiazepine Symposium (TIBS) in September 2017.

Most of 2016 was spent planning the TIBS event. I had no idea my notion of an educational conference on benzodiazepines would require so much.

We hired a medical director, recruited speakers from around the world, and complied with the requirements to offer Continuing Medical Education (CME) credits to the registrants.

Friday, September 15, 2017
The International Benzodiazepine Symposium

The day has arrived!

The speakers came from near and far – Ireland, Massachusetts, California, to name a few. The Keynote Speaker was none other than Robert Whitaker, whom I had tracked down at the Empathic Therapies Conference two years earlier.

Over the three day event we heard from experts on sleep, stress, trauma, and research.

We discussed addiction and recovery with a focus on healing.

The intention for the Symposium was to issue a call for further evidence based research into benzodiazepines and other bio-psychiatric medications. Please understand we are not out to "bash benzos", we are aware of their potential positive use in traumatic situations.

We are not in support of castigating or litigating against the pharmaceutical companies. However, we do support legislation protecting patients with "Advised Consent" information.

I believe our intention was well received and the energy at the Symposium was productive.

Speakers and attendees alike seemed excited and eager to take our message forward.

Epilogue

"I know what I have given you. I do not know what you have received."
— ANTONIO PORCHIA

There you have it. One woman's ten year tale through the labyrinth of Benzomania, finally emerging whole again and with new intentions.

Have I furthered your knowledge about this "invisible brain disorder"?

Would you like to support an online Hotline for people in the throes of withdrawal?

Would you like to see a benzodiazepine withdrawal and recovery treatment home in your state?

Would you like to get ads for bio-psychiatric drugs off the TV and out of magazines?

Will you warn people you know who are dealing with anxiety to look at the information presented herein?

Perhaps you have ideas for other ways to combat this "benzo scandal" that has become a catalyst for profit, rather than well-researched and healing.

Where we go from here will depend on how we advocate for next steps to assist in recovery and prevention.

Using restorative practices and inviting the Pharma Lobby to work with us is one of the ways to create new prescriptions for benzodiazepine reform.

I invite any pharma representative, retired or active, to join us in finding the keys to recovery for the millions of patients still suffering in silent agony.

Each of you comes in contact with folks who have been inadvertently caught in the benzo trap I crawled out of in time to rebuild my life. The brain is a forgiving entity, We do heal! Make sure everyone knows this.

All Because of My Precious Granddaughter

Why undertake this passion to write about Big Bad Pharma and how it continues to capitalize on the blunting of billions of brains? You can blame it on my now almost six year old granddaughter, who is growing up in a culture with the belief that there is a pill for just about anything that troubles you; a culture of addicts, former addicts, damaged people doing damaging things.

Before this precious little girl entered my life – making me a grandma for the first and only time – I didn't have to worry about the next generation being handed an ailing society and planet.

I will be thrilled if *Repairing the Benzo Blunder: A Mosaic of Recovery...*
  - hits a nerve somewhere in a system that has been so ravaged by ignorance and greed.
  - causes one CEO of one of the companies that manufacture psychoactive drugs to consider helping patients shift from benzodiazepines to alternative plant-based calming protocols and behavioral therapies.
  - educates about the benefits of close attention to restorative nutrition and disciplined daily exercise.
  - helps even one person ask the questions about benzodiazepines I did not know to ask.

Even more important, I want to affirm that my granddaughter and her generation will not be victimized by pharma-experimentation and exploitation.

Instead, they should grow up making informed choices in a benzodiazepine blunder-free world.

— MARJORIE MERET-CARMEN

Acknowledgments

No one writes a book like this alone – though this one began in a very solo moment one afternoon in 2012 when I just about ran my car off the Bill Healy Bridge in Bend, Oregon, on my way home from yet another puzzling doctor's appointment.

No, this ten year personal and spiritual odyssey into and finally out of "benzo-madness" would not have found its way into print without the assistance of many mentors and my editors who took the roughest of first drafts, and like a clump of clay, sculpted this mosaic of memories, research-based conclusions, journal entries and poetry into *Repairing the Benzo Blunder: A Moasic of Recovery*.

Along the path to what now feels like a miraculous recovery, the list of those who lighted my way included: Professors Malcolm Lader and Heather Ashton, Robert Whitaker, Geraldine Burns, Monica Cassani, Jim Dobbins MP, Barry Haslam, Baylissa Frederick, Holly Hardman, David Healy MD, Peter Gotzche MD, Laurie Iriland, Luke Montegu, Gwen Olsen, Jack Stein PhD, Steve Wright MD, Howard Zehr, Greg Morris, Ellen Waterston, Louise Hawker, Thomas Osborne, Peter Wilberg, Kristi Miller, Lisa Denhem, Crystal and Daniel Wright, and Ray Nimmo.

Antonio Porchia

I would be remiss if I neglected to mention how the poetry of Antonio Porchia helped me through the dark days and nights. I gleaned solace from his wisdom.

Porchia (1885-1968) was an Argentinian poet. An influential, yet extremely succinct writer, he has been a cult author for a number of renowned figures of contemporary literature and thought. I include quotes from *Voices*, a translation of Porchia's work by W.S. Merwin, throughout the book.

AfterWords

The AfterWords section includes a lengthy list of resources and communications with leading benzo authorities. This is more than just a compendium of citations. For the benzo-dependent, their families and support networks these resources provide valuable information regarding the "how to" of recovery.

I have worked to verify accuracy of all the information and quotes in this book. However, please note that I gathered many of these references while my brain was still healing. It is important to understand that our individual brains are a different configuration of synapses and DNA material specific to each of us. I do not represent myself as a medical expert, nor am I qualified or intend to deliver any medical diagnosis or prognosis. Again, I encourage everyone to do their own research and come to their own conclusions.

1. Iatrogenesis: inadvertent and preventable induction of disease or complications by the medical treatment or procedures of a physician or surgeon. Merriam-Webster.com, https://www.merriam-webster.com
2. Mandorla: Wikipedia, https://en.wikipedia.org/wiki/Vesica_piscis
3. Lewy Body Dementia: www.lbda.org/category/3437/what-is-lbd.htm
4. https://www.ncbi.nlm.nih.gov/pmc/articles/PMC3939441/Patients who undergo anesthesia and surgery appear to have nearly a two-fold increased risk for dementia, new research shows.
5. Ashton, Heather. "Benzodiazepines: How They Work and How to Withdraw" http://www.benzo.org.uk/manual/
6. http://benzobuddies.org an Anonymous Benzodiazepine recovery forum.

7. Tolle, Eckhart. Popular spiritual author in the U.S. https://www.eckharttolle.com/.

8. Lane, Christopher. "Brain Damage from Benzodiazepines: The Troubling Facts, Risks, and History of Minor Tranquilizers." Researchers have long known that benzodiazepines can cause brain damage. Side Effects, *Psychology Today*. November 18, 2010.

9. http://www.independent.co.uk/life-style/health-and-families/health-news/ drugs-linked-to-brain-damage-30-years-ago-2127504.html

10. Whitaker, Robert. *Mad in America: Bad Science, Bad Medicine, and the Enduring Mistreatment of the Mentally Ill*. Basic Books; 2 edition, May 25, 2010. In addition, Robert Whitaker notes in his 2010 book, *Anatomy of an Epidemic: Magic Bullets, Psychiatric Drugs, and the Astonishing Rise of Mental Illness in America,* Crown, April 13, 2010. that in 1983, "The World Health Organization noted a 'striking deterioration in personal care and social interactions' in long-term benzodiazepine users." (Whitaker, 138). More recently in 2007, he continues, "French researchers surveyed 4,425 long-term benzodiazepine users and found that 75 percent were markedly ill to extremely ill...a great majority of the patients had significant symptomatology, in particular major depressive episodes and generalized anxiety disorder, often with marked severity and disability (Whitaker, 137).

11. Resources for these teachers can be found at www.soundstrue.com

12. Frederick, Baylissa. *Recovery and Renewal: Your essential guide to overcoming dependency and withdrawal from sleeping pills, other 'benzo' tranquillisers and antidepressants.* Jessica Kingsley Publishers; Revised edition, May 21, 2014.

13. Neale, Greg and Smith, Allan J. "Self-harm and suicide associated with benzodiazepine usage," The British Journal of General Practice. May 2007.

14. Hollis PhD., James. *Swamplands of the Soul: New Life in Dismal Places (Studies in Jungian Psychology by Jungian*

Analysts). Inner City Books. First Paperback Edition, September 1, 1996.

15. For more information on Malcom Lader visit http://www. benzo.org.uk/lader2.htm

16. https://www.benzo.org.uk/lader6.htm

17. Gershon, Michael. *The Second Brain: The Scientific Basis of Gut Instinct and a Groundbreaking New Understanding of Nervous Disorders of the Stomach and Intestines*. Harper, 1998.

18. For more information on GABA, visit McGill University's site, The Brain From Top to Bottom. http://thebrain.mcgill. ca/flash/d/d_04/d_04_m/d_04_m_peu/d_04_m_peu. html

19. For more information on Reg Pert visit http://www.benzo. org.uk/peartbio.htm

20. Levine, Stephen. Loving Kindness Meditation.

21. Estes, Marla. Making the Unconscious Conscious: Embracing the Dark Night of the Soul. https://beyond-meds.com/2013/04/17/embracing-the-dark-night/

22. Campbell, Joseph. *Reflections on the Art of Living*, Diane K. Osbon, Editor. Harper Perennial. Reprint, May 1995.

23. The Role of GABA and GABA receptors in benzodiazepine withdrawal, http://www.benzosupport.org/gaba.htm

24. Purgatory: https://www.britannica.com/topic/ purgatory-Roman-Catholicism

25. Goldacre, Ben. *How Drug Companies Mislead Doctors and Harm Patients*, Farrar, Straus and Giroux; Reprint edition, April 1, 2014.

26. The Cloud of Unknowing is an anonymous spiritual guide on contemplative prayer written in the latter half of the 14th century. The underlying message of this work proposes that the only way to truly "know" God is to abandon all preconceived notions and beliefs or "knowledge" about God and be courageous enough to surrender your mind and ego to the realm of "unknowingness," at which point, you begin to glimpse the true nature of God.

27. Hawryluk, Markian, "Benzodiazepines treat anxiety, cause long-term problems." *The (Bend) Bulletin*, June 3,

2014. I was featured in this article about long-term benzo use. http://www.bendbulletin.com/home/2119922-151/benzodiazepines-treat-anxiety-cause-long-term-problems

28. The hypothalamic-pituitary-adrenal (HPA) axis is a complex set of interactions between the hypothalamus (a part of the brain), the pituitary gland (also part of the brain) and the adrenal or suprarenal glands (at the top of each kidney.) The HPA axis helps regulate things such as your temperature, digestion, immune system, mood, sexuality and energy usage. It's also a major part of the system that controls your reaction to stress, trauma and injury. Research links fibromyalgia and chronic fatigue syndrome with abnormalities in genes involved in the HPA axis. The HPA axis is also involved in anxiety disorder, bipolar disorder, post-traumatic stress disorder, clinical depression, burnout and irritable bowel syndrome. It was once thought that the brain sends out these "information substances" to respond to problems in the body and that the communication was one way. But it is now becoming clear that the CNS controls the body's defense mechanisms. Knowing this, we can assume that every thought, emotion, idea or belief has a neurochemical consequence. https://en.wikipedia.org/wiki/hypothalamic-pituitary-adrenal_axis

29. http://www.coptic.net/EncyclopediaCoptica/

30. https://archives.drugabuse.gov/sites/default/files/monograph33.pdf

31. https://www.benzo.org.uk/appg23-10-13.htm

32. Dr. Leo Sternbach is credited with creating Valium. http://www.benzo.org.uk/valium2.htm

33. http://www.empathictherapy.org/Founding-Guidelines.html

34. Breggin, Peter R. *Your Drug May Be Your Problem, How and Why to Stop Taking Psychiatric Medications*, Da Capo Lifelong Books; Rev, Upd edition, July 10, 2007.

35. Royal College of Psychiatrists: http://rcpsych.ac.uk/discoverpsychiatry/thepresidentsblog/internationalcongress2015.aspx

36. All quotations from Professor Ashton used with her prior consent.
37. http://www.benzo.org.uk/profash.htm
38. http://advocateforsocialreform.com

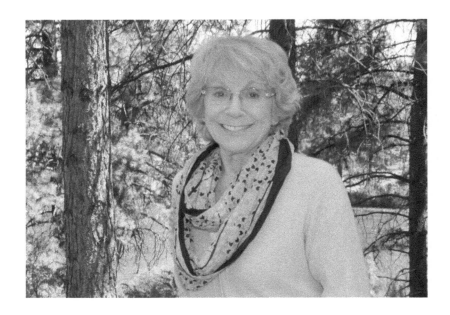

About the Author

Marjorie Meret-Carmen, M.Ed. is an educator, freelance writer and social and political activist. She wrote *Repairing the Benzo Blunder: A Mosaic of Recovery* during her ten-year dependency and ultimate recovery from a benzodiazepine (Ativan), prescribed during her husband's long neurological decline and subsequent demise.

As the founder of Advocates for Social Reform, Marjorie is committed to finding solutions to social issues that have been plaguing society for centuries.

Marjorie Meret-Carmen earned a Master's degree in Education from Antioch University in 1979.